Stability for Seniors

Discover the Secrets of Posture, Balance and Stability in Your Golden Years

I0435424

RON KNESS

CONTENTS

INTRODUCTION

Did you know that 7 out of 10 seniors have stability issues and actually fear they will lose balance and accidentally fall? To some, the fear of falling may seem trivial. Yet to the 65+ age group, the thought of falling can be a stressful thing. Many seniors fall each year and the results can be devastating. Hip fractures are the worst; many never fully recover and end up in an assisted living facility.

Studies show that people who fall during their senior years are much more prone to injury and sometimes even death.

Many older people wonder if it's possible to improve their balance and also get stronger so that they'll be more stable. Should they accidentally trip or slip, their bodies would be more resilient and they will be able to handle the impact.

This is a sensitive topic and definitely warrants much attention. The hard truth is that people do not become physically unstable or unbalanced as they age. Of course, there is no denying that a certain degree of strength and mobility is lost.

However, the main reason people become frail and weak is due to a lack of exercise. This may seem unpalatable because it highlights one's neglects and failings. The truth is bitter.

You may have noticed that some people in your neighborhood, who are in their 60s, have trouble walking and getting around. Yet, if you look at Sylvester Stallone, he is still muscular and in excellent shape. He is still directing and getting physical in his action movies. Stallone is in his sixties.

What about Arnold Schwarzenegger? His arms and muscles are bigger than those of men half his age. He doesn't seem to lack coordination or balance.

The dancer, Michael Flatley, is 57 and still dancing. The former model, Christie Brinkley, is sixty and she is as elegant and fit as ever.

What is the underlying reason here? Why these people are healthy and well-coordinated while you or others you may know are sickly, unfit or unable to move without assistance?

The answer is – the life choices we made.

Many people sacrifice their health in pursuit of their career. They are so busy making a living that they neglect to make a life. The excuse that they do not have time to exercise is tossed about so frequently that they end up letting their health and fitness slide.

If you are not regularly active, you will have muscular atrophy over time. Your flexibility will decrease. Your core strength will diminish. As time progresses, you will be less limber and more rigid.

This is exactly how people age poorly. It's a process that has snowballed over time.

Only with regular exercise and a healthy diet can you have a body that is fit and has the ability to almost reverse aging.

Dan Inosanto, is 79 years old and he is still fit and active. He used to train Bruce Lee and many other martial artists. The martial arts are one of the best forms of exercise.

Why?

Because you need balance, flexibility, strength and stamina to excel at it. All the punching, kicking and movements will help the body to retain its natural vigor and vitality.

If you have neglected your health for years and life seems to be a chore now because you can't get around without assistance, do not feel dejected.

You can remedy the situation. You can restore the strength, balance and stamina that you have lost. It is never too late to become what you might have been. Your body will help you, if you help it.

This guide will show you exactly what you need to do to restore your balance, strengthen your core and give you the ability to live life to its fullest. Read on…

CHAPTER 1 – Why Do We Fall?

Before even looking at how to prevent falling, you will need to understand why older people are more prone to falling. You must understand the root cause of the problem before you seek the remedy.

There are several possible reasons why a person may fall. Let's look at some of them.

Loss of traction/footing

The ground could be slippery leading to a loss of traction. This often happens in bathrooms where the floor is slippery.

This can easily be solved by placing an anti-slip mat on the floor of the bathroom. In fact, it his highly recommended that all seniors place these mats around the base of their toilets or bathrooms.

Even with a strong core and good stamina, if the floor is slippery, there is really nothing much you can do to prevent a fall. The best you can hope for is to fall the best you can to avoid major injuries. Try to not break your fall with your hands as that is a leading cause of broken wrists. If you know you are going to fall, try to roll once you hit the floor.

Tripping

Another reason for falling is tripping. People have tripped over carpets, children's toys, shoes, table legs, stools, etc. My wife tripped because the sole towards the toe on the bottom of her shoe had come loose, hooked on something and down she went. Fortunately she did not get hurt.

Always keep your home tidy and organized. Make sure your carpets do not get in your way when walking. If the sole of your shoe is starting to loosen up, get a new pair.

If you have grandchildren, get them to store their toys away after play. If you use the staircase at home, always have one hand on the handrail and always be careful.

Prevention is better than cure. Being mindful of where you are going and what you are doing is the first line of defense against falling.

Aging

The third reason is aging. Yes... we have to admit that things generally slow down as we age. One important thing that slows down is our reflexes. When you're young, your responses are much faster and swifter.

If you trip, you instinctively reach out to grab something to stabilize yourself. If you slip on a slippery surface, your feet may make a few quick backward steps to compensate and regain your balance.

When you're old, before your instincts and reflexes can kick in, you're already on the ground. Your reaction time will be much slower when you're old. Regular exercise and sports can improve your reflexes.

Vision problems

Vision problems are another often neglected issue. Many accidents have taken place on the road involving seniors who are pedestrians. They're often unable to see the traffic lights or the oncoming traffic clearly.

In the home, they may not be able to see objects in their way and may trip on them. Using spectacles may help but if the glasses are bifocal, there may be depth perception issues that could pose possible problems.

In cases like these, it's best to keep the surroundings at home clear, easily navigable and well-lit. Most falling incidents happen at home.

Muscle atrophy and strength loss

As a person ages, there is a change in the body's composition. People are more prone to weight gain and muscle mass decreases. In fact, men lose 1% of muscle every year from the age of 30.

This is why regular exercise is so crucial. It cannot be overemphasised. Only regular exercise, especially weight training, can retard muscle loss. In fact, it can even cause muscle gain. And the more muscle you have, the more calories you'll burn – even while at rest. Why? Because the more muscle mass you have, the more calories it takes just to keep the muscles functioning.

Strong leg muscles and a strong core will prevent people from falling. Imagine a tree... your legs are like the roots and your abdomen (core) is like the trunk. If these are strong, the tree won't fall... you won't fall. That's really all it is in a nutshell.

CHAPTER 2 – Who Is Most Likely to Fall?

There is no particular age group or sex that is exempt from falling. Anybody can fall at any time regardless of age or gender. However, since this guide is focused on stability for seniors, we'll look at who is most likely to fall in this age group.

Whether a senior is more predisposed to falling is predicated on a few factors. We already looked at why people fall. Now let's look at who is most likely to fall.

Older people

The older you get, the more likely that falling becomes a possibility. People in their seventies are at greater risk than those in their sixties. Those in their eighties are more prone than those in their seventies and so on.

The reason for this is that we get weaker as we get older. Exercise will mitigate most problems but we must be realistic. The type of exercise you do as you age will change dramatically. Someone in their eighties will probably benefit most from walking and light weight training.

Forget the CrossFit, HIIT and strenuous exercises. Most people will not be able to handle these training methods in their golden years.

People with Chronic medical conditions

Unfortunately, as people age, the immune system gets weaker and many people get afflicted with health issues that take a negative toll on their health.

In some cases, the condition is so bad that the person affected is in bed most of the time. At times like these, due to inactivity, muscle mass decreases and they get weaker.

Once they get up from bed, their legs and the core stabilising muscles may be weak too. These conditions increase the tendency of falling and it's essential to have a caregiver present to prevent an unfortunate accident from occurring.

Fogginess, dizziness, disorientation, poor blood circulation, etc. are all common side effects of chronic illnesses and the fact that seniors are older, exacerbates the situation. All these directly or indirectly may result in falling.

Generally, as people age, they lose their fat stores too. The soles of the feet that used to be cushioned are now bony and painful. Walking becomes a chore and standing can be tiring and painful. With less cushioning on the feet, the impact from walking resonates throughout the body. This too can cause a loss of balance.

CHAPTER 3 – Am I Susceptible to Falling?

This is an excellent question. It shows that you're proactive and interested in your well-being. Many people automatically resign themselves to their problems and blame it on aging. The first step in prevention is in being aware of your situation.

One thing that I have noticed is that I'm more unstable first thing after getting up in the morning. Once I have taken a few steps, I'm fine. I have never fallen (yet), but I'm fully aware of my situation so I'm super careful.

There are a few questions you will need to ask yourself before you can ascertain if you might fall. Of course, even if the answers indicate that you don't, you may still fall. Life can be unpredictable and anything is possible.

However, for the most part, the questions below will give you a good idea of your chances of falling.

Have you been physically active for most of your life?

If you have been exercising daily or frequently all throughout your life, your body will be stronger and more coordinated than someone who has led a sedentary life all the way into their senior years. Your chances of falling will be lower.

Are you still exercising now?

Some people exercise for most of their life but taper things down and stop as they get older. They either lose interest, motivation or they just give up.

You must carry on exercising and tailor your workouts to suit your lifestyle. Generally, your training should be lower impact and at a slower pace. There is no shame in slowing down. It does not matter how slowly you go, as long as you do not stop.

If you're still getting regular exercise, your chances of falling are lower.

What type of exercise do you do?

The type of exercise you do will also determine your chances of falling. Not all exercise is created equal. If all you do is a slow walk for 30 minutes every morning your chances of falling will be higher than someone who does Pilates or weight training regularly.

Why?

Because with Pilates and weight training, the core muscles and other important muscles are worked. The stronger your muscles are, the more optimally the body functions as a whole.

Stronger legs mean that you're more capable of walking, running, climbing stairs, etc. You may have noticed that many seniors have problems going down stairs. It's often more difficult than climbing stairs.

The reason for this is the flexors in the legs are used when climbing stairs and are generally stronger. Extensors are generally weaker and recruited into action when descending stairs.

If you have worked the extensors during strength training with lunges, Bulgarian split squats, etc. your legs will be stronger and you will be less prone to falling.

Muscle memory

If you were a dancer, gymnast, martial artist, etc. in your younger years, the body would have developed an innate sense of balance that never really goes away. Your chances of falling will be much lower.

There is no denying that what you do when you're young directly impacts your condition when you're older. Aikido is a Japanese martial art and its masters are usually well into their sixties.

They have been practicing the art for years and their bodies move gracefully and have developed the reflexes and 'flow' that can only come from a lifetime of training. They're often much better at the art than people much younger than them.

This is proof that you can retain your mobility, balance and strength even as you age.

Consuming Alcohol

If you consume alcoholic beverages, your chances of falling will be much higher. This is true whether you are young or old.

Your reflexes slow down, you get sleepy, disoriented and lightheaded. All these can cause you to fall. Exercise due caution if you're drinking... and always drink in moderation.

CHAPTER 4 – Beginning the Road to Recovery/Instabilityy Prevention

First and foremost, you must understand that no matter how weak you think you are or how inactive you have been, you can ALWAYS improve your situation.

Never underestimate the power of small positive daily action that snowball over time. There are people in their sixties who started going to the gym and ended up with bodies that are better than the majority of people half their age.

Consistent and conscientious action is a force to be reckoned with. Before looking at the road to recovery or instability prevention, let's look at the consequences that can occur should you fall.

This may seem scary to some but it's important to know the possible scenarios that can result when a senior falls down for whatever reason.

Dislocation/Fractures

This is one of the most common scenarios that occur when a senior falls. Unlike younger people who are more resilient and can handle the impact, older people usually have more brittle bones.

Some may even suffer from osteoporosis. The fragility of the bones poses a huge risk during a fall. Fractures can easily occur since the bones are less dense.

It's easy to dislocate a shoulder or a hip during a fall. It all depends on the force and the direction of the fall. Either way, it's not a pretty scenario.

Death

This is a very real possibility. There are thousands of documented cases of seniors who have died from a fall at home, either in the bathroom or by tripping on the stairs. They may hit their head and never regain consciousness, or fall and can't get up. If there is no one that regularly checks on them, they end up dying of dehydration.

If you live alone, subscribe to some type of medical alert service, such as Life Alert at http://lifealert.com – the "Help, I've fallen and I can't get up" people.

By the way, I have no connection or receive any commission from them; I just know they are one of the best companies in this business.

Most of them give you a little device that you can wear on your wrist or around your neck, so if you fall, (and stay conscious) you can press a button and they will send help.

It is not a pleasant thought but we must stare the hard facts and once we know what we're looking at, we can take steps to prevent the worst from happening.

Now let's look at how we can begin on the road to recovery.

Committing to exercise daily

This is the first and most crucial step. Just like with weight loss, a commitment is required. You must have a plan and stick to it. Unlike with weight loss, your training sessions will be much shorter and less strenuous.

The goal here will be to increase the strength of your core muscles, stabilising muscles, flexors and extensors. You will also need to increase your flexibility in order for your joints to be more supple and limber.

Get your vision checked

This is the second step. If your vision is fine, that's excellent. No further action required. However, if your vision is not good, you should get glasses or whatever you need to see well.

Get good footwear

It is perfectly normal for older people to have less cushioning on the soles of their feet. It would be an excellent idea to get a pair of sports shoes with good cushioning that you can wear at home. Make sure the soles have good friction with the ground. This will reduce any chances of slipping.

Now, not only do you have good support but you've reduced your chances of an accidental fall. Two birds with one stone. Excellent.

Get Your Blood Pressure Checked

It's quite common for older people to have a drop in blood pressure when they stand up. They might feel lightheaded or giddy. While these are usually short spells lasting for 10 to 20 seconds, the risk of falling is high. So, it's best to be cautious and check your blood pressure when you're seated, lying down and standing.

Know the Side Effects of Your Medication

Are you on medication? Do any of the medicines you consume make you drowsy? Even normal cold medication that makes a younger person drowsy has a much more soporific effect on an older person. The side effects are multiplied due to the weakened state of the person as they age.

Once you discover which medications are making you sleepy or drowsy, you should ensure that after consuming them, you're either in bed or comfortably seated and maybe watching TV.

Do not consume medication and go out to do gardening or try to play with your grandchildren. You must be ever watchful and mindful of your actions.

Eliminate Hazards at Home

Rearrange your furniture if you have to. Make it easier for yourself to move around in your home. Sacrifice decor and ambience for pragmatism and safety.

Improve the lighting in your home. Make sure that items that you frequently need or use are within reach. Do not store important items in high cabinets that will require you to use a foot stool to reach.

Ideally, you should not use ladders, stools, boxes, etc. to reach higher places. Err on the side of caution. Get someone to help you when you need it. Relinquish the need to show how independent you are. People will help you if you need help.

Install handrails or grab bars wherever you need them. Even mountain climbers usually try their best to have 3 points of contact at all times. It's all about balance and being secure.

CHAPTER 5 – What Sort of Exercise Should I Do?

In this chapter, we will look at the different types of exercise you should do to improve your balance, stability, strength and stamina.

This is the most important chapter in the book. Read it and re-read it to fully understand what you need to do. As long as you adhere to the points in this chapter, you will drastically reduce the chances of you falling.

Work on Your Stamina

When you were younger, you could easily go for a run or a jog. You might have been out of breath after a while if you were not in shape… but you'd still be able to do it.

However, when you're much older, running or even jogging may not be an option for you. If you've been a runner or jogger all your life, you will still be able to do it when you're old. If you've not, it will be a Herculean task. Most people will just not be able to do it.

So what should you do?

You should walk. This is one of the best forms of cardiovascular training for older people. The reason cardiovascular exercise is so important is because it keeps your heart healthy and gets your blood flowing. It will boost your blood circulation tremendously.

You could start with a 10 minute walk and increase it to 20 minutes until finally you can do it for 30 minutes. You really do not need to go on longer for 30 minutes. The goal is to get these 30 minutes of exercise daily.

Usually, in your senior years, you will have a lot of time. The overused excuse of not having time to exercise no longer applies. Ensure that you walk daily.

Aim to increase your speed over time. Brisk walking is very beneficial. Gandhi used to walk 11 miles daily and called it the "prince of exercises". Brisk is defined as having an elevated heart and breathing rate, but still being able to carry on a conversation while walking.

Other types of cardio that you may do are swimming, stationary bike, rowing machine, etc. Do note that cycling on a stationary bike is very different from cycling on an actual bicycle. It is not recommended for seniors to ride a bicycle.

Even if you're perfectly able to cycle, there is always the off-chance that a dog or child may get in your way and you may lose control of the bike and fall.

Stick to safe activities.

Core training

Two of the best forms of core training are yoga and Pilates. If you can find Pilates or yoga classes near you, check if the instructor is able to accommodate an older person in their class.

In almost all cases, the instructors will be extremely helpful and glad to help someone who is making an effort to learn. That's just the way it is.

Cast your fears aside and join these classes. Your flexibility and core strength will build up over time. Time is your greatest ally.

Since these are low impact exercises, you will not be breathless. You should progress at a pace you're comfortable with. If it hurts, don't push it. Tell your instructor what you can do and what you're having difficulty with.

Pilates was created by Joseph Pilates to rehabilitate soldiers who were injured or maimed. It will definitely help you increase your flexibility, strength and stamina.

Initially, it may seem intimidating to do Pilates or yoga. Some seniors may find it too tough. Rest assured that you only need to do what you can and over time as you get better, you will be able to handle the more advanced poses.

Ask your instructor to create a program that you can handle. Practice makes perfect. Make measurable progress in reasonable time.

What if I Can't Join a Pilates or Yoga Class?

If you can't join these classes, there are a few exercises that you can do that will achieve similar goals. The key is to do them daily. In some cases, you can split your sessions throughout the day.

For example, you could spend your morning doing about 15 minutes of stretches and in the evening you may do strength training. There are no hard and fast rules here. You must listen to your body and do what feels comfortable.

If you do not know what the exercises are below, you can always Google them or check on YouTube for video demonstrations.

Core training at home

Planks

One of the best exercises for abdominal core training is planks. These are far more effective than sit-ups and crunches. They involve much less movement but are just as effective.

There are a few types of planks (with a YouTube.com reference on how to do each move), such as:

- Elbow planks
  (https://www.youtube.com/watch?v=K-DBIY19KW8)
- Plank Up-downs
  (https://www.youtube.com/watch?v=L4oFJRDAU4Q)
- Side Planks
  (https://www.youtube.com/watch?v=z4DjimUbvGc)
- Top of push-up planks
  (https://www.youtube.com/watch?v=o2Qek4N2ea8)
- Spiderman planks
  (https://www.youtube.com/watch?v=HVyHcalg61g)
- Side plank – knee to elbow
  (https://www.youtube.com/watch?v=6VCUrTHEqgg)
- Plank walks
  (https://www.youtube.com/watch?v=pF19C4Xq_Rs)
- One-leg plank
  (https://www.youtube.com/watch?v=Nlu0vWJhss8)
- Reverse plank
  (https://www.youtube.com/watch?v=STCe7-aZ-o8)

- Bird dog
  (https://www.youtube.com/watch?v=wiFNA3sqjCA)
- Floor bridge
  (https://www.youtube.com/watch?v=lkYUwiKSEmI)

As long as you do the plank exercises above, your core will be strong. You do not need to do them all in one day. You can do 2 or 3 a day and change them up on different days.

The key is to hold the plank for as long as you can. Despite the fact that not much movement is involved, these are very challenging exercises and you will find your body trembling and you may even be sweating and panting.

Do not push yourself too hard but do challenge yourself a little. Always use a yoga mat. This extra bit of cushioning will make it easier on your palms, elbows and knees. You can also use rolled up towels or small cushions under your elbows if they hurt.

Strength Training

This involves working with weights or your own bodyweight. Initially when you're starting out, you can just stick to bodyweight training.

In fact, if you do not wish to go beyond bodyweight training, that's perfectly fine. However, many men who do get into strength training may find that they could do much more in a gym. It's totally your choice though.

Let's look at some of the best bodyweight exercises.

- Standard Pushups
  https://www.youtube.com/watch?v=Eh00_rniF8E

- Wide-grip pushups
  (https://www.youtube.com/watch?v=G05EwTHYxLU)
- Narrow grip pushups
  (https://www.youtube.com/watch?v=G2mlaEfpEIM)
- Single leg pushups
  (https://www.youtube.com/watch?v=RO8pcUwLl28)
- Burpees
  (https://www.youtube.com/watch?v=tJrdJBWBu08)
- Squats
  (https://www.youtube.com/watch?v=nEQQle9-0NA)
- Lunges
  (https://www.youtube.com/watch?v=QF0BQS2W80k)
- V-sit
  (https://www.youtube.com/watch?v=I_1KGrBx2T4)
- Toe stands (*Hold the back of a chair for support and slowly stand on your tiptoes*)
- Knee curls (*Hold the back of a chair for support and just curl your knee backwards*)
- Leg straightening (*Sit upright on a chair and straighten your leg. Hold for as long as you can and lower it. Repeat as many times as you can for both legs*)

Using weights

If you do not wish to go to the gym, you can get a set of dumbbells and do arm curls, side arm raises, elbow extensions, etc. All these are resistance training exercises that are very effective.

As long as you do the exercises mentioned earlier, you will be just fine. They're low impact but very effective for building strength and muscle.

CHAPTER 6 – Stability Training Methods

Just by working on your strength and stamina as mentioned in the earlier chapter, your overall stability will improve by leaps and bounds. However, there is one last side to this triangle… and it is flexibility.

All of us lose flexibility as we age. That's why we are more prone to strains, pulls, muscle tears, etc. The key to avoiding all these issues is to stretch for 10 to 15 minutes daily. There is no need to aim for the splits like, Van Damme, does… but you should still stretch to stay limber. With each stretch below is a YouTube reference on how to do the stretch:

- Neck rolls
  (https://www.youtube.com/watch?v=yMJcEukHtnA)
- Arm rotations
  (https://www.youtube.com/watch?v=i1_Vn6XyORk)
- Shoulder rotations
  (https://www.youtube.com/watch?v=uFnx9sA_LCs)
- Knee rotations
  (https://www.youtube.com/watch?v=MXe0DS51MY8)
- Ankle rotations
  (https://www.youtube.com/watch?v=exR-hiMGQDM)
- Yoga sun salutation
  (https://www.youtube.com/watch?v=uMV4Nq6jpu0)
- Standing side to side bends
  (https://www.youtube.com/watch?v=4TSmAsa8FPc)

- Calf stretches – standing calf stretch, wall stretch (https://www.youtube.com/watch?v=JSzCfi0wbcA)
- Hamstring stretches (https://www.youtube.com/watch?v=C-wiOqYcxoI)
- Cat-camel backstretch (https://www.youtube.com/watch?v=CXRsjICsGnc)
- Squat stretch (https://www.youtube.com/watch?v=oWe37lYEWZg)
- Seated forward bend (https://www.youtube.com/watch?v=HyiFhjwWXkw)

If you have postural problems that are causing pain in your back or hips, you will need to seek the help of a medical professional. Usually these are chronic and in some cases people might have nerves that are pinched resulting in severe pain (i.e. sciatica). Get professional help as soon as you can.

CHAPTER 7 – Stability Supports

In this chapter we will look at the different types of stability supports available to you should you need one.

Before looking at what products are available, we will need to address the elephant in the room… and that is the major shift in mindset that is required.

There are thousands of seniors who vehemently refuse to use walking canes or braces. They feel that it makes them look handicapped or worse… like an old person.

Getting old is as much a mental game as it is a physical one. This is especially so for people who led active lives and slowly find that as they age, their strength and speed is diminishing. This can be depressing to say the least.

They feel like it's an insult and a sign of helplessness to use assists. The need to appear strong and independent is so great that they're willing to endure life with much struggle.

The truth of the matter is that a walking cane is not a sign of weakness. You cannot afford to have this mindset. Walking aids are designed to help you. Using one effectively and helping yourself is a sign of strength and independence.

If you need one, get it… and use it. Never ever regret growing old. It is a privilege denied to many.

The best person to speak to in regards to using walking aids will be your doctor. If your problem is due to a lack of strength, you could make your muscles stronger and the problem would resolve itself.

However, if the issue is due to something else that can't be resolved and your only option is a walking cane, then you will definitely need to get one. Your doctor will be able to tell the difference and let you know if you really need a cane or not. Of course, ultimately, the choice will be yours.

Now let's look at the different types of walking aids.

Walking canes

We all know what these are. They're usually made of aluminum with one end being a handle and the other having a rubber tip. Some walking canes are adjustable (about 33 to 37 inches) and some are foldable for convenience. When choosing a cane, make sure it is sturdy, yet lightweight and easy to carry.

Walkers

These provide more support and balance than canes. However, there is a certain social stigma to using these and many older people prefer walking canes because they're less obvious.

Seniors who are weaker and unable to stand for long would be best off using walkers.

Most walkers are foldable and have 2 wheels in the front (about 5 inches in diameter) which are fixed.

Mobility scooters

These are usually the most convenient and the issue of falling while walking becomes moot because you're seated and zipping around from point to point. The only downside is that they can be pricey. However, this is a one-time investment that will pay dividends many times over in terms of convenience and safety.

CONCLUSION – How to Begin the Road to Recovery or Prevention Today

The very fact that you've made it to the end of this guide shows that you're willing to see things through to finality. This is an excellent trait to have and will serve you well in your recovery.

Now that you know what to do in terms of training and requirements, you will be better prepared to help yourself regain your balance and stability.

Always remember that Rome wasn't built in a day. It will take time for your body to adapt and get stronger. You will need to be patient and consistent. It is the consistent daily effort that matters. Like Buddha said, "A jug fills drop by drop". There is no need to rush.

Make a plan and stick to it. If you commit to 15 minutes of exercise daily, then stick to it. Try out all the different exercises mentioned so that your training has variety and you're targeting different muscles. Aim for small incremental improvements in your performance.

Follow the precautions mentioned in chapter 4 closely to reduce any chances of you falling. You can never be too safe.

Last but not least, stay positive and do not feel depressed about aging. Have a sense of humor. Like Bob Hope, said, "You know you're getting old when the candles cost more than the cake." Be proud of your achievements and that you have made it this far. Age is just mind over matter. If you don't mind, it doesn't matter.

"Aging can be fun if you lay back and enjoy it." – Clint Eastwood

Other Senior Health and Fitness Books by This Author

If you would like to read more about Senior Health and Fitness, here is a list of the <u>titles, CreateSpace links and descriptions:</u>

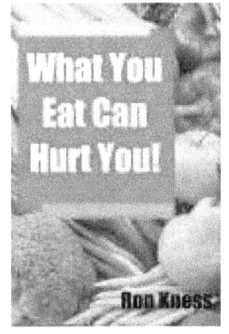

What You Eat Can Hurt You

https://www.createspace.com/4963196

Do you know that certain foods increase your risk for inflammation, disease and illness? It's true! And certain foods can help cure and heal you if you do get sick. Knowing which foods to eat and which ones to avoid empowers you to manage your own health.

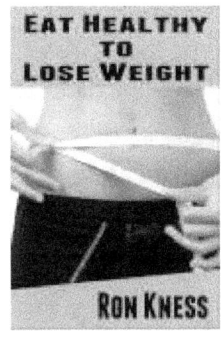

Eat Healthy to Lose Weight

https://www.createspace.com/4962939

As you read through our book, we show you which foods you should and should not be eating to reach your weight loss goal, along with discussing how to maintain your weight loss and stay within a few pounds of your goal weight. Banish the weight you keep gaining back each time by learning how to live a healthy lifestyle.

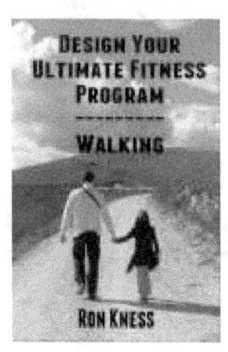

Design Your Ultimate Fitness Program - Walking

https://www.createspace.com/5252272

In my book Design Your Ultimate Fitness Program – Walking, we discuss the considerations that need to be made when designing a custom walking program, along with:

• Equipment needed
• Wearable technology you can use to track your walking
• And how to make walking more challenging

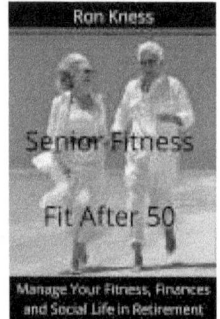

Senior Fitness – Fit After 50: Learn How to Manage Your Fitness, Finances and Social Life in Retirement

https://www.createspace.com/5474751

Inside you will discover answers to your most pressing questions:
• What do I need to know about downsizing my home?
• What are the best tips for staying healthy as you approach your 50's?
• When should I start planning for retirement?
• I am worried about being lonely once I retire, do others feel the same?

• Is it worthwhile to carry two homes during retirement?
And more…

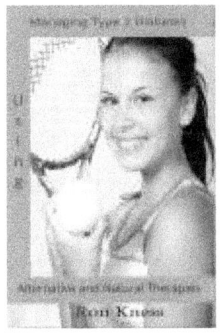

Managing Type 2 Diabetes Using Alternative
And Natural Therapies

https://www.createspace.com/5401244

While Type 2 diabetes can be managed
medically, there are many alternative natural
and holistic methods of therapy and treatment
that can further enhance quality of life and
minimize the effects of this disease. In this book, I discuss 12
different types, including yoga, reflexology and acupuncture to
name just three.

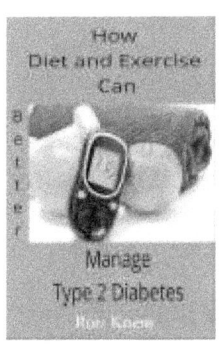

How Diet and Exercise Can Better Manage
Type 2 Diabetes

https://www.createspace.com/5404845

Of the different types of diabetes, only Type 2
can be reversed. In my book How Diet and
Exercise Can Better Manage Type 2 Diabetes,
we reveal the three things you can do to best
manage your disease, including:
• Diet
• Exercise
• Weight management

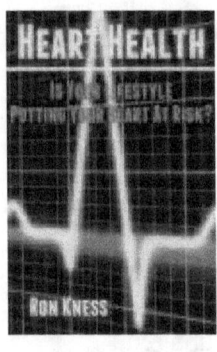 Heart Health: Is Your Lifestyle Putting Your Heart at Risk?

https://www.createspace.com/5464020

In my ebook Is Your Lifestyle Putting Your Heart At Risk? we discuss the six greatest risks to your heart and the lifestyle changes you can make to mitigate them.

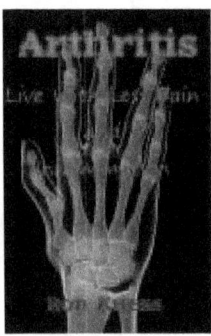 Arthritis – Live Wth Less Pain and Inflammation: Tips and Techniques You Can Use to Lessen the Pain and Inflammation

https://www.createspace.com/5457441

Discover Simple Tips & Information That Will Help Reduce The Painful Symptoms Of Arthritis!

You learn things like:
• Simple and effective information that will help you manage the pain and inflammation that comes along with arthritis, so that you can live an active, full life without debilitating pain.
• The different types of arthritis, their symptoms and how to alleviate their painful side effects.
• The pros and cons of over-the-counter arthritis medications, plus simple tips that will help you know how to choose the right supplements.
• Free, yet effective ways to get relief from arthritis pain and inflammation, so you don't have to suffer anymore.

the effects arthritis can have significant impact on your physical and mental well-being, but this books shows you how to overcome its painful symptoms and live life relatively pain free.

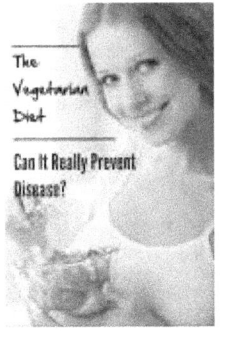

The Vegetarian Diet – Can It Really Prevent Disease?

https://www.createspace.com/5519874

Is a vegetarian diet right for you? Multiple studies have shown over and over that a vegetarian diet goes along way in preventing certain chronic diseases, such as:

• Heart Disease
• Cancer
• Diverticulitis
• Type 2 Diabetes
• Hypertension
• Obesity
• Kidney Failure

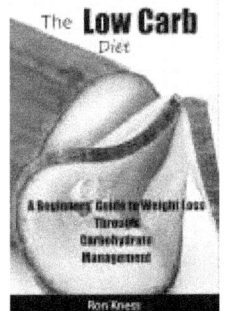

The Low Carb Diet: A Beginner's Guide to Weight Loss Through Carbohydrate Management

https://www.createspace.com/5416348

In my book "The Low-Carb Diet – A Beginners' Guide to Weight Loss Through Carbohydrate Management", I reveal a successful method of losing weight based in part on the amount and type of carbohydrates you consume.

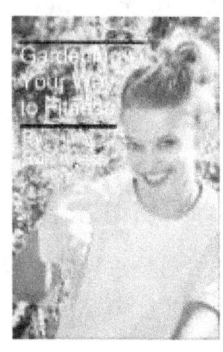

Gardening Your Way to Fitness: The Fun Way to Get Fit and Provide Beauty and Healthful Bounty for Your Family

https://www.createspace.com/5459564

The gym is a great place to stay fit during the colder seasons, but once the temperature turns warmer you want to spend more time outside. Plus, you'll have the benefit of fresh wholesome produce to enjoy by growing vegetables in your backyard garden.

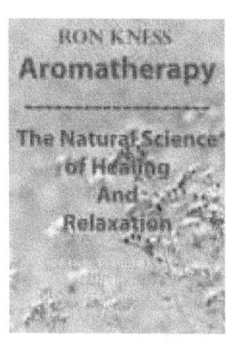

Aromatherapy - The Science of Healing and Relaxation: Learn How Essential Oils Elicit The Relaxation Response And Alter Mood

https://www.createspace.com/5714434

In my book Aromatherapy – The Science of Healing and Relaxation, we reveal the natural holistics methods you can use to heal the body from certain medical issues and to relive stress through relaxation. In particular we talk about:
• Aromatherapy - what it is and how it works
• Essential Oils – how the effects of certain aromas differs from others
• Recipes – how to make your own essential oil combinations

ABOUT THE AUTHOR

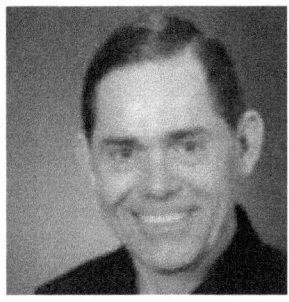

I grew up in Central Minnesota, where my parents own and operated a fishing resort. Once out of high school I tried a couple of semesters of college, only to quit halfway through the Spring term; I decided at that time that college wasn't for me.

Then I decided to follow my father's previous occupation as an auto mechanic. I graduated from a two-year of vocational training course and worked as a mechanic. While in vocational training, I decided to join the National Guard where I eventually ended up working full-time for 32 years.

So how does all of this relate to writing? In one of my leadership schools, the instructor, who was an English teacher at a juvenile detention center, presented writing to me in a whole new way - a way that started to develop my interest in working with words.

Fast forward about 40 years and I now have over 50 books listed on Amazon for Kindle and CreateSpace.

www.ingramcontent.com/pod-product-compliance
Lightning Source LLC
Chambersburg PA
CBHW071310280526
45788CB00004B/1872